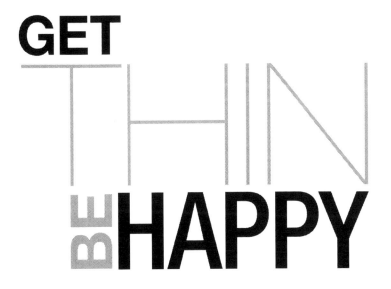

GET THIN BE HAPPY

The Six Easy Steps to
Becoming Thinner,
Healthier, and Happier

BRYAN D. TODER

Published by:

Wizard Marketing Corp.
P.O. Box 94
Eagleville, PA 19408-0094
USA

GetThinBeHappy.com

To my mother, Gwen,
who's funnier than she thinks.

To my father, Ellis,
a genius inventor who never stops thinking.

To my sister, Randi,
whose potential is endless.

Disclaimer

This book has been written to provide instruction in learning how to reduce the fat in your body in order to lose weight. Every effort has been made to make this book as complete and accurate as possible. However, there may be mistakes in typography or content.

The purpose of this book is to educate. The author and publisher do not warrant that the information contained in this book is fully complete and shall not be responsible for any errors or omissions. The author and publisher shall have neither liability nor responsibility to any person or entity with respect to any loss or damage caused or alleged to be caused directly or indirectly by this book.

Legal Notice

This book is designed to provide information in regard to the subject matter covered. While attempts have been made to verify information provided in this publication, neither the author nor the publisher accept any responsibility for errors, omissions, or contrary interpretation of the subject matter.

This information is sold with the understanding that the publisher and author are not engaged in rendering medical, psychological, or other professional services. If medical or other expert assistance is required, the services of a competent professional should be sought.

The publisher wants to stress that information contained herein may be subject to varying state and/or local laws or regulations. All users are advised to retain competent counsel to determine what state and/or local laws or regulations may apply to the user's particular business.

The purchaser or reader of this publication assumes responsibility for the use of these materials and information. The content of this document, for legal purposes, should be read or viewed for entertainment purposes only.

Adherence to all applicable laws and regulations, including federal, state, and local, governing professional licensing, business practices, advertising, and all other aspects of doing business in the United States, or any other jurisdiction is the sole responsibility of the purchaser or reader.

The author and publisher assume no responsibility or liability whatsoever on behalf of any purchaser or reader of these materials.

The publisher will not be responsible for any losses or damages of any kind incurred by the reader, whether directly or indirectly arising from the use of the information found in this book.

This book is not intended for use as a source of medical, psychological, legal, business, accounting, or financial advice. All readers are advised to seek services of competent professionals in the medical, psychological, legal, business, accounting, and finance fields.

The reader assumes responsibility for use of information contained herein. The author reserves the right to make changes without notice.

The sole purpose of these materials is to educate and entertain. Any perceived slights to specific organization or individual are unintentional.

The testimonials used in this book are from past clients of Bryan Toder.

Contents

Foreword.. 9

About The Author 12

Acknowledgments 13

Introduction... 14

Part 1: Diet And Exercise.............................. 16

Diets— Why They Won't And Can't Work 19

    But, I've Lost Weight By Dieting In The Past! 19

    Homeostasis Or The Set Point 20

Exercise—"Do I Have To?!" 22

    So, Why Do I Need To Exercise? 22

    What Happens When You Exercise?...................... 24

    Other Benefits 24

Part 2: The Lose Weight— Be Happy! Program 27

What To Expect.. 29

    Change Is Good, But Fast Change Is Bad.............. 29

    How Will You Know This Is Working?...................... 30

    Confidence And Sabotage...................................... 31

    You're Going To See Small Successes 32

    Relax And Have Fun... 33

The Lose Weight—Be Happy! Six Simple Steps

To Losing Fat... 34

    Step One: Eat To Get Thin 34

    Step Two: Get A "B" 37

    Step Three: Enjoy It 100 Percent!........................... 38

    Step Four: Know When To Stop Eating 39

    Step Five: Exercise Consistently 42

    Step Six: Water, Water, Water 44

    A Review... 46

Part 3: Reprogramming Your Life 48

Why You Do What You Do 51
    Pain And Pleasure 51
    A Sharp Stick 51

Last On The List 53
    Savior To Your World 53
    Put Yourself First 54

Changing Your State 58
    Special Bonus! 59
    About Hypnosis 60
    Emotional Eating 62
    Physiology? 62
    Goals And How To Meet Them 63

Special Bonus Section 65

Linking Pleasure To Exercise 67
    Creating The Motivation To Exercise 67

Your Compelling Future 70
    Trouble Visualizing? 72

Controlling Cravings 73
    Creating A Resource State And Anchoring It 73

Fixing Your Self-Image 75
    The "Thinner You" Mirror 76

Questions And Answers 79

Final Thoughts 89

Additional Resources 91

Foreword

Are you excited to leave struggle, diets, sacrificing and deprivation behind? What a wonderful journey—from fat and frustrated to thin and satisfied... happy with how you look, fitting into the size of clothes you've had in mind and feeling great about yourself!

Congratulations on picking up this book; it's a wonderful resource for you, written by a trainer who is one of the elite experts in weight-loss. And a bigger congratulations for living your life by design and choice, making the commitment to take a little better care of yourself and get healthy.

What you're about to learn may be a different way of thinking about weight and health (and what's possible) than you've done before. And that's a good thing. The weight-loss industry has been misleading and disappointing people for years and the information you now have is the way out of all that useless dieting thinking and failure.

The real bottom line issue with excess weight is actually pretty simple. You're overweight because you're using food to change how you feel. You want to go from stressed to calm, or anxious to relaxed, or maybe even bored to not bored, and food has become the way you calm down or feel differently.

Now that's actually a big concept, and it starts to explain why diets fail ninety-five percent of the time. You're not overweight because you haven't counted enough calories, or measured enough fat grams. In fact, naturally thin people don't obsess about those sorts of things. Nor do they get on the scale very often. The weight problem that has kept you feeling depressed, anxious, sad, frustrated and even guilty is actually controlled in your unconscious mind as a way of distracting you from emotional stress or discomfort. It is the right-brain, unconscious mind-controlled, emotionally-based behavior that can begin your change immediately. *How exciting is that?!*

Since all habits and your emotions are controlled in your unconscious mind (and hypnosis deals exclusively with the unconscious mind) you can start to notice that the "fix" for the problem is exactly where the problem is in the first place—in your unconscious mind. So with the help of hypnosis, you're in the right place to change things.

Bryan is a master at helping people tap into the power of their unconscious mind to easily and almost effortlessly create the kinds of changes in their bodies, thinking and self concepts they have longed for. Many clients find that the side benefits of hypnosis—such as profound relaxation and calmness and better confidence and security about themselves—are even more valuable than the actual weight loss they first came for.

Your journey into health and fitness will be unique to you, of course, but know that you are about to begin a fun and fascinating time where you can truly make the kinds of changes that you only imagined.

Good luck and have fun! You're about to find out you deserve to be happy and you *can* change your life.

— **Julie Nise, MA, LMT, LPC, CH**
    Licensed Marriage and Family Therapist
    Certified Hypnotist
    Southeast Hypnosis Training Institute
    Author of *4 Weeks to a Happier Relationship*

About the Author

Bryan Toder is a professional clinical and certified hypnotist at *Plymouth Hypnosis Center* in Lafayette Hill, Pennsylvania.

Bryan began his career performing stage hypnosis, and in 2001 he branched out from stage hypnosis to clinical hypnosis where he helps clients conquer their fears, manage stress, quit smoking, and, yes, lose weight.

As a master hypnotist and master practitioner in Neuro-Linguistic Programming (NLP), Bryan also teaches people to change their lives for the better.

And, he's an entrepreneur who markets information—an infopreneur. At GetThinBeHappy.com, Bryan helps others to learn how to lose that excess fat—*the easy way!*

Note: If you have any questions or need help with the concepts taught in this or any of our informational books or e-books, feel free to drop Bryan a line at www.GetThinBeHappy.com/contact

— Bryan D. Toder
GetThinBeHappy.com

Acknowledgments

This book would never have been possible without the mentorship and friendship of Dr. Scott McFall whom I met in 2000 in order to learn Clinical Hypnosis.

Scott has guided me throughout these years to create a hypnosis business at *Plymouth Hypnosis Center* that has helped thousands of people change their lives for the better.

Without Scott's help, the ideas in this book would never have been possible.

Introduction

Bob came into my office tipping the scales at 425 pounds. He, like, I am sure, all of you, tried to lose weight with dieting, but, in Bob's case, this always caused his gout to reoccur. Nothing worked and his own doctor was throwing his hands up. Bob mentioned hypnotism to his doctor who said, "Well, why not?"

Today, Bob is over 200 pounds lighter! Then, in his "self-improvement" mode, he got Lasik eye surgery, new front teeth, and a wonderful life. When we were talking years later, he told me, "For the first time in my life I can sit in my chair at home, and my little dog can sit next to me." Wow.

It took about four months for Susan, a physician, to reach her weight-loss goals—and remain there. Like many of you, she had failed in the past, but, Susan was able to, finally, lose weight and become a comfortably thin person for the rest of her life.

After just six weeks of hypnosis with me, Paul's doctor reduced his diabetes medicine. He's now totally off his blood pressure meds, too. His weight is coming off slowly but regularly. Like most of my successful clients, he's healthy and happy.

As you know, The United States (and most of North America has a real weight problem. Since the 1990s, Americans, even though they're living longer, have been getting bigger and unhealthier.

Heightened diabetes rates, knee replacements, increased stress, cancer, back problems, heart disease—the list is almost endless because Americans are getting huge. This has got to stop. You *can* do it.

What my clients have taught me is what this amazing program to reprogram your mind, become healthy, lose weight, and get happy is all about!

— Bryan D. Toder
June, 2010

P.S. I titled this book *Get Thin—Be Happy!* This doesn't mean that you can't be happy if you are not thin; that would be absurd. It only means that many, many people would and could lead a happier life if they lost the unnecessary weight in their bodies. Generally, you'll be healthier—and happier—in the long run!

For additional information and updates to this book, please go to www.GetThinBeHappy.com.

PART 1:
Diet and Exercise

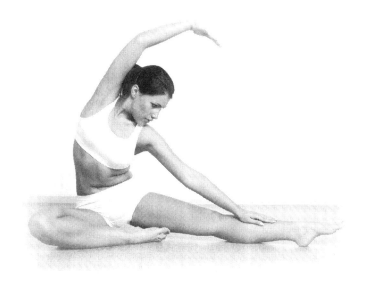

Diets – Why They Won't And Can't Work

Diets—they're everywhere: on television, bookshelves, magazine covers. Promoted by movie stars, famous singers, soap opera stars—even the "ordinary mom"— these fad diets are prolific. Literally thousands and thousands of new diets promoted every year!

And *none of them work.* Period.

"Really?!" you ask. "None of them?"

Yes, none. How do I know this? Because—and really think about this—if even *one* of those fad diets actually worked… *it would just work!* Not for a few, but for just about everyone. And not for only a few weeks or months either.

But, I've Lost Weight By Dieting In The Past!

Uh huh. Yes, you can *temporarily* lose weight. Fine. However, permanent weight loss cannot be achieved by dieting. (No, not even dieting *and* exercise, but that's later in this book.)

You See, What Happens With The Typical Dieter Is This:

- You realize you need to go on another diet.
- Next, you find a diet and begin.
- Deprived of food, you lose some weight.
- Your metabolism slows down *because your body needs food!*
- Loss of essential muscle tissue occurs, and, since

muscle weighs more than fat, you lose some more weight.
- Continuing to eat less food, your body adjusts its metabolism rate—its set point or homeostasis—again. New food gets stored as fat.
- Now, your body is starving. Really, it is starving.
- You become tired and lethargic. (Maybe even a bit cranky!)
- Something happens. Stress, an office party, the smell of lasagna… and you crack!
- You begin to eat the way you did before the diet, but since your metabolism has been slowed, most food that you eat gets stored as fat!
- You feel like crap and eat more and …

Sound familiar?

Homeostasis Or The Set Point

We all have a set point, or homeostasis, of where we should be weight-wise. This is primarily determined by age, activity, and food intake.

The set point influences the food you eat and your appetite. Decrease your eating and your body slows down to protect its fat stores. In other words, eat less, burn less.

You start to lose energy and slow down. You move less and less. Exercise is a chore. Your body loses muscle tissue and reduces the metabolism again.

Now, your body is responding differently to how it uses insulin and that causes you to, yes, store more fat!

What you need to do instead of just looking to eat less is to restore the right level of homeostasis and live a healthier life.

Fortunately for you, this set point can be changed and *you* are in control of it!

Exercise – "Do I HAVE To?!"

Of all things, my weight-loss clients just love to exercise. Some of them just can't wait to jump out of bed, drive to the gym, and workout …

I can't even type that with a straight face.

Okay, most of them *hate* it. They hate exercise or have no motivation to exercise or it hurts or whatever weenie excuse they have for not doing it that day.

But, exercise is 100 percent essential for your success in weight loss. Without it, you're only half-baked.

Later in this book, we'll discuss exercise in more detail, but why do you need to exercise at all?

No, weeding your garden is *not* exercise.

So, Why Do I Need To Exercise?
Change That Set Point
Exercise changes the homeostasis set point. It's that simple. And to do this, the exercise must be consistent.

So many of my clients would explain that they had exercised two or three days in the week since I last saw them. And they were proud of it.

Now, when one begins an exercise program, beginning at two or three days a week if you've not exercised regularly for a long while is a good start. However, to lose fat and keep it off, one must exercise at least six days a week for at least forty minutes a day. No excuses. To lose fat, you'll need to exercise.

This will also increase your metabolism which will burn off more fat!

Increased Muscle

Exercising, especially strength training with weights or bands, is wonderful. You will add a nice layer of muscle (lean body mass) to your body and this will increase your metabolism. Yes, you may actually gain weight by doing this and this is typical and it is why, as you will see later, you won't be using the scale to determine your success.

By adding that nice, healthy muscle and increasing your metabolism you will actually burn fat while resting. Even while you are sleeping! Exercise is looking better, isn't it?

Cardio exercise is great, but it's a better idea to incorporate strength training with the cardio. As I heard one trainer say, "If you're pear shaped to begin with and you only do cardio, you'll just be a smaller pear."

One of the things I hear from my female clients is that they're afraid that, by exercising—especially strength training, they will "bulk up" and get too muscular. Let me assure you that, unless your diet includes anabolic steroids, and I'm quite sure it doesn't, that won't happen.

It can't. Don't worry about it.

By doing strength training you will reshape your body. Men will look muscular and women will look sexy. (And, you'll be able to wear those sexy dresses you've been afraid to wear!)

What Happens When You Exercise?
(This is fascinating ... *really!*)

You can *only* lose fat by burning it off with exercise. Remember that. You burn off fat in the muscles.

And, the more muscle you have, the more fat-burning enzymes you'll produce. *Why do you need the enzymes?* Read the next part. You'll love this.

Here's What Happens During Exercise:
- Exercising starts a process where fat molecules leave the fat cells.
- *If you have enough muscle* and if your muscle needs energy and it has the fat-burning enzymes, then the fat molecule will move to the muscle and burn off!

That's how you burn fat.

Of course, if you don't have enough muscle tissue, that fat molecule will wander around and return to its fat storage cells. Nothing happens and you stay fat.

Additional information about exercise and fat burning can be found in an amazing, hard-to-find book, *How to Lower Your Fat Thermostat* by Dennis W. Remington, Edward A. Parent, and A. Garth Fisher.

Other Benefits
Of course, being "in shape" with exercise has some added benefits!

First, you'll look better. Clothes will fit the way they should and you'll look great.

Second, you'll feel better. Seriously, lose even ten pounds of fat and your whole body will thank you. If you need to lose thirty or more, and do so, your body will feel young again.

Third, you'll be stronger. You can do things that weren't possible before — like playing a sport, running with your dog, or lifting your child or grandchild!

Fourth, you may live longer. You may reduce the possibility of diabetes (or if you have it already, you may become healthier), lower your blood pressure, lower cholesterol, and take the weight off your knees and back. (Check with your personal physician before changing any medications!)

And more. The actual benefits of exercise are almost endless. Just do it.

"I have lost over 30 lbs. and no longer have high blood pressure. I find it easier to not think about/crave unhealthy foods."

— Veronica Katz

"I've taken a variety of steps to lose weight and had successes, but found that each time I would slip back into a different mode and regain the weight.

"This method with Bryan seems different. The weight loss has been gradual and comfortable and it feels more like a lifestyle change than a diet."

— Dr. Joseph Nines, Psychotherapist, lost over thirty-five pounds.

PART 2:

The Get Thin— Be Happy! Program

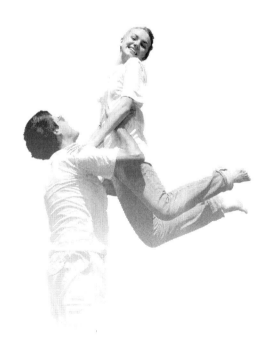

What To Expect

It never fails to amaze me how quickly my weight-loss clients want to get results. Yes, I can hypnotize someone to quit smoking in one easy session, but you don't need cigarettes to live! (You still need to eat, right?)

It took you a long time to put that weight on. It will take some time to get it off.

Change Is Good, But Fast Change Is Bad

The body hates change. If one loses a leg, the body is "searching" for it; it believes it's still there. It's still trying to pump blood into that area and it's in shock. This, by the way, is why liposuction is somewhat of a questionable procedure. Your body is instantly losing the fat it is used to having. Suddenly, it's gone! Not a good thing.

Women who give birth find that their body still thinks it's pregnant. It's still producing hormones and it wants to hold onto the same weight (homeostasis).

Now, you may not want to hear this, but the *best* way to lose weight is *slowly*. You kind of need to "sneak" it off your body. If you try to lose weight too quickly (crash diets, starvation, etc.) your body will fight to keep the same weight. If you lose weight slowly, it "gets used to" the new weight set point.

So, the first thing to expect is slooooow results. Expect it.

This, however, does not mean that you can't lose ten or so pounds in little more than a week; it just means *don't put any pressure on yourself to lose weight in a short time.* You aren't in a race, are you?

How Will You Know This Is Working?

Easy—you will be measuring yourself every *six weeks*. Yes, six weeks. Oh, and *no scales* ... promise?

Why?

Two reasons:

First, your weight does not show your success. You can gain weight by eating a meal or lose weight by going to the bathroom.

Second, it's discouraging. Jumping on and off the scale is what overweight people do. Naturally thin people, for the most part, do not care what they weigh; they care how their clothes fit and how they look and feel.

So, think like a naturally thin person and stop weighing yourself.

Measuring

You will measure yourself in a few areas and with different methods. First, get your body fat tested and write it down. You'll want to have this tested every sixty days or so.

Next, you'll measure several areas, write them down, and measure again every *six weeks*.

Measure your neck, upper arms (at the bicep), chest (across the nipple area), waist (across the navel), hips, and thighs.

You will find amazing results every six weeks and you'll be very proud of yourself. So, no weighing, okay?

Realize, the *Get Thin—Be Happy!* Program is really about fat loss, not just weight loss. Yes, you'll lose weight, but stop focusing on it for now.

Confidence And Sabotage

Sure, you've tried a bazillion other ways to lose weight and failed at all of them. (If you lost weight and gained it back, that's a failure.) So, what makes you think that the *Get Thin—Be Happy!* Program will work?

Because it's not your diet and exercise drivel. It's a lot more. It's about reprogramming your mind.

However, we need to talk about two things: confidence and sabotage.

Confidence

Just decide to "keep the faith" and "stay the course." If you follow the very simple steps outlined in this book, you should reach your goals!

Sabotage

Yikes! Sabotage—from others or even *you*—can destroy your momentum. Just be aware of the possibilities of people sabotaging your new success. "Oh, honey, have some dessert. You can eat better tomorrow." Or, "You look great just the way you are!" (This is usually said by someone who wants you to stay fat—*sabotage!*)

Just be aware that it exists—even from the people who love you the most.

Use these negative people to help you succeed by saying

this to yourself whenever you receive a negative comment:

"Each negative person or comment around me just reminds me to live a thin lifestyle."

Oh, and if you screw up … just start again from where you are now. *Remember, you only lose if you quit. Don't quit—stay the course.*

Watch Out For Indifference

Have an absolute conviction that you will succeed. Indifference is the killer of success, and it is caused by an unwanted belief that you cannot succeed. If you can't succeed, then why try? This is what most people think. (You don't want to be like most people.)

Recognize indifference for what it is. Thoughts like, "This won't work," "I'll never succeed," or "No one will believe I can do this, so I'll just quit" are ludicrous.

Combat indifference by doing something positive to reach your goal. Even if you have little, tiny successes you will chip away at indifference.

You're Going To See Small Successes

One of the wonderful things about the *Get Thin—Be Happy!* Program is the chance to succeed in small ways. Again, you won't be losing a huge amount of weight like on a crash diet where you'd gain it all back—and more! You'll see and feel things in the next six weeks like:

- Your clothes will fit better.
- You'll have more energy.
- People will comment on how relaxed and calm you

are.

- You'll sleep better.
- You may receive some comments about how "different" you look.
- You'll feel more "in control" of food, your appetite, and our body.
- And *more!*

Relax And Have Fun

Just give the *Get Thin—Be Happy!* Program a chance. Relax in the realization that you can succeed! Just have fun with this.

The *Get Thin—Be Happy!* Six Simple Steps To Losing Fat

The thing I find funny about the *Get Thin—Be Happy!* Fat-Loss/Weight-Loss Program is that people expect it to be so painful and difficult. In fact, I am convinced that the very notion that this program is so easy to do sometimes allows them to think that nothing that's too easy can actually work. ("If it was so easy …" Finish the sentence yourself.)

Conversely, if it was difficult to do, then the excuse would be that it was "too hard." Of course, you just can't please everybody.

The *Get Thin—Be Happy!* Program is easy, it works, and it's fun. So, just do it and forget the excuses, okay?

Step One: Eat To Get Thin

What?! Eat and get thin? *What kinda cockamamie idea is that?*

Like I wrote in the first section of this book, you will need to eat. I bet, like most people, that you don't eat enough or often enough.

Are You One Of Those People Who...
… skips breakfast?

… eats on the run?

… has lunch at your desk and takes bites between tasks?

... snacks between meals so that you don't pass out from hunger?

... has a huge dinner because you are just starving?

... snacks from dinner until bedtime?

If you do even one of the events above, you aren't eating enough or often enough.

Think about it, if you were a prisoner and you were given just a bit of food—every so often—would you eat it all at once? Maybe, but more than likely, you'd hide it away for later. That's just what your body does when you are starving it. Yes, by eating like the above examples, you are starving yourself.

Your body is very, very smart. It knows exactly what to do to survive—*in spite of what you do to it.* So, realize that when you starve your body it will store the food—as *fat.*

Fat, as you may know, is how your body stores its food. It creates fat storage for those times when it needs food or extra energy, like when you exercise.

Eat too much and the excess food gets stored away. To make matters worse, if your metabolism is slow, as it probably is now, it can't easily burn off the excess fat. Even worse, when you don't eat enough, the metabolism slows down even more. And, around and around you go into a spiral of getting fatter and slowing down your metabolism.

So, What's The Solution?
Eat when you are hungry.

Let me get a little specific here and say that I don't mean

when you just want "something crunchy" or "something sweet"… I mean *hungry*.

I don't mean when you are *starving*. I mean:

When you feel you need to eat—eat!

Here's a sliding scale for you to determine your need to eat:

How Hungry Are You?

1. Starving
2. Headaches and Feeling Faint
3. Very Hungry or Famished
4. **Somewhat Hungry**
5. **Not Hungry at All**
6. **Satisfied with What You've Eaten**
7. Full
8. Stuffed Like a Turkey
9. Painful & Hard to Move
10. Sick & Nauseous

Ideally, you should only be in areas four to six. If you wait until you are very hungry (three), it's getting to be too late. Eat. If you wait until one or two, you'll be at the mercy of anything and it could make you sick.

Stop eating when you are satisfied. This is Step Four of the *Get Thin—Be Happy!* Program and six on the above chart.

Rule of Thumb: Never get below four or above six.

Portion Sizes

Just a side note about portion sizes. My clients learn the best way to eat is using portions, and it's a simple, easy formula:

A protein (poultry, beef, pork, fish) the size of the *palm* of your hand.

A complex carbohydrate (brown rice, 100 percent whole wheat bread, potato, etc.) the size of your *fist.*

A vegetable a few times a day. (You know what a vegetable is.)

How Hard Is That? Easy, Right?

At home, portion it out and put the food away. Don't just leave it out for you to munch on. Portion out the food, eat, and you're finished.

At a restaurant, if you get a huge dinner, just portion it out. Box up the rest (right then and there) and eat what's left.

You can do it.

Step Two: Get A "B"

Do you want to succeed at this? Just do this program correctly 85 percent of the time and you should succeed.

That's a "B," people. Get a "B" at this and you should lose the desired fat and weight.

So, if you're at your kid's birthday party and you want a slice of cake … eat the cake. *But, enjoy it 100 percent!*

If you're at the movies and you want a bag of popcorn,

get a small bag (without the butter, okay?) and *enjoy the popcorn 100 percent!*

If you want _____—eat it, *and enjoy it 100 percent!*

Step Three: Enjoy It 100 Percent!

Steps Two and Three are joined at the hip. Eat what you want, but only if you enjoy it 100 percent. The moment you are thinking that you're done—*stop eating immediately.*

If you're having that popcorn, for instance, the moment you are not enjoying that popcorn to its fullest, stop eating. That's pretty easy, right?

What I Learned At A Buffet

A few years ago, I was hungry and stopped by a Chinese buffet near my office. For $6.35, you could eat all you want. So, I grabbed my dish and put a few items on my plate and sat down.

As I was eating I noticed that most of the patrons were grossly overweight and I made some observations:

- These people were in a hypnotic trance! (I noticed they were staring at a spot while eating.)
- They ate and ate and ate without really enjoying it—almost mindless (like when you eat a snack while watching TV).
- They all had way too much food on their plate. This is a result of what's called "Poverty Consciousness." This has nothing to do with how much money one has; it's the thinking one has when "I don't know if I'll ever eat like this ever again!"

(This happens at a wedding, on a cruise, buffets, etc.) Remember, you can always get food, okay?

The conclusion I came up with was that these people have completely *disassociated* from their bodies. As if they were a head with feet with nothing in between. (And, if you were grossly obese would you want to associate with your body? Your mind is very powerful and protective.)

The only time when they feel full is when it's way too late. They are stuffed.

Too Late — Stuffed Like A Turkey!

Perhaps, the same thing happens to you at Thanksgiving dinner. You're eating your meal, talking, and listening to stories… and eating. You're disassociated from your body and the meal, distracted by the festivities.

Then, you might take seconds and continue what you've been doing.

Then—you notice your clean plate and ask yourself about… *thirds?* That's when you do what naturally thin people do all along; *you check to see if you are full.* And, what happens? You immediately feel overstuffed, bloated; you unbutton your pants, pat your stomach, and it starts to hurt.

It's too late. The meal is ruined. What a night!

So, how do you fix this?

Step Four: Know When To Stop Eating

As I alluded to above, naturally thin people constantly check to see if they are full. And, when full, they stop.

Kids Do It Naturally!

Ever see a child eat? When they are done, well, they're done! "I'm finished. I'm not hungry! I don't *want* anymore!" They push their plate away *because they know they are full.*

So, what does the parent (or grandparent) say? "Eat it or no dessert for you!"

The Guilt

Remember this one? "Think of all the starving children in Asia! You'd better eat!
Finish everything on your plate!"

(I remember as a child wondering if anyone really shipped their half-eaten roast beef to the Far East. I mean, *how is that done?*)

This, of course, is why you feel so guilty about leaving food on your plate. Fortunately, the self-hypnosis program (see Appendix) you get for free with this book will help you with the childhood guilt associated with not "cleaning your plate."

Know When To Stop Eating — The Steps:

This is a very easy way to relearn how to feel full. The same way children and naturally thin people do it!

Step 1: After you put the food in your mouth, eat slowly and chew your food completely.

Step 2: Remember, you must enjoy the food 100 percent or stop eating!

Step 3: Go "inside" and check to see if you are full. Now, of course, in the very beginning you won't feel full, but you need to get into the habit of checking. So, go "inside" (in hypnosis terms that means to feel where the food is) and check. Are you full?

Step 4: If not full yet, keep eating.

Step 5: Repeat Steps one through four.

By constantly checking over and over, putting your utensils down and enjoying your food 100 percent, you will notice exactly when you're coming up to the "full" point.

Step 6: When full, *stop eating.*

That's how naturally thin people—and now, *you*—eat!

Note: Most people eat too quickly. Take small bites and chew your food completely. It will take about twenty minutes to get the "full" feeling so give yourself the time to get that feeling. Eat slowly.

Here's a Funny Thing That Naturally Thin People Do Too:

When choosing what to eat or while looking at a menu, naturally thin people determine what they want to eat *by imagining what it would be like to have already eaten that meal.*

They look at the meal and think, "How would this feel in my body after I've eaten it?"

Will you feel bloated, too full, greasy, heavy, or light?

For example, if you're going out dancing after dinner, would eating spicy Indian food really be a good idea?

Step Five: Exercise Consistently

Yes, as you read in Part One, exercise is *essential* for this to work. If you skip this step, you're only doing part of the plan.

The hardest part of exercise for most people is finding the time. I hear this daily in my hypnosis clinic. "I just don't have the time."

But, the time is there; it just needs to be managed. The best time to exercise is just after you wake up, before you begin your full day.

Brush your teeth, get on your exercise clothes, and begin.

Do You Need A Gym?

I personally exercise at home. Why? Because it's quick, easy, cheap, and I don't have to impress anyone.

When I went to a gym it to took way too long:

- Ten minutes to the club.
- Ten minutes to check-in, get to the lockers, and change.
- Two hours to work out because I had to wait for machines and it was crowded.
- Twenty-five minutes to shower, change, and get to my car.
- Ten minutes to home.

That, people, is almost three hours to work out! No wonder most members quit within their first month at a health club.

When I need to exercise at home, if it's a forty-five-minute workout, it takes fifty-five minutes if you include the shower.

So, forget the fancy clubs. Save your money and stay home.

Good Exercise

So, what should you do? If you don't have any medical issues or a bad back or knees it's suggested that you begin with *brisk* walking. Walk twenty minutes a day for a week. Each week increase your walk by five minutes until you are walking briskly for an hour a day.

If it's too cold, snowy, raining, too hot… whatever, then go to a local mall and walk. If you have to, walk up and down your hallway.

Do whatever it takes.

This is where most people create excuses. Make that appointment with yourself to exercise. Don't wait until you get home or "later" as it'll never get done. Just do it.

Then, start a strength training program. Dumbbells, exercise bands, and a chair are all you need for most programs.

I would suggest buying a DVD on this. Go you your local sporting goods store and ask for a suggestion. Not bodybuilding—exercise with dumbbells and/or exercise bands. For about seventy-five dollars you can get a good set of dumbbells or bands.

Exercise at least *six* times a week for optimum fat burning.

Out Of Shape?

If you are so out of shape that even walking is out of the

question, start small. Sit in a chair and stand up. Then sit down. Do this several times. Take a break and repeat. Do what you can.

Will this burn fat? Not yet. This is to start exercising and get you used to moving. Some people almost never move; this is just to get you used to it. Then, when you are ready, start with the walking described above.

Note: Be sure to check with your personal physician before beginning any exercise program of any kind.

Step Six: Water, Water, Water

Do you know those ads for those "famous" weight-loss or diet centers where they have testimonials like,

"I lost ten pounds in fourteen days at _____ Weight Loss"?

Did you ever wonder why you hear this so often? It's because of water!

It wasn't the amazing weight-loss center or their magical scales or the "delicious" meals they tell you to buy (costing you around $5,000–$6,000 a year!). It was the water they drank. Lots and lots of water.

You (yes, you!) probably don't drink enough water. Most people don't, and you need to.

Why? Because you need to metabolize the fat in your body.

One of the main functions of the liver is to convert stored fats into energy. But, if the kidneys are not getting enough water to work properly, the liver will need to step in and pick up the slack—which takes away from its main function, converting that fat into energy.

So, drink less water and store more fat. It's an easy equation.

"But, This Is Too Hard To Do!"

One of the easiest ways to lose about ten pounds is to start drinking water. *Is that really so hard to do?* Of course, you'll be running to the bathroom constantly, but after a few weeks your body will become accustomed to the water and you won't be running so often.

This is because your body will not have to retain the water anymore because it "knows" that it'll get hydrated! (Your body is very smart.) You see, your body was in "survival mode"—it didn't know when or if it was going to get its necessary water. So, after a week or so, the water it had been retaining is flushed out of the system. (This is usually eight to ten pounds of water!)

Some Additional Benefits To Drinking Water

Did you know that drinking eight to ten glasses of water a day will also help you look and feel younger?

Drinking water will:

- Flush out impurities in your skin.
- Improve your complexion.
- Hydrate your skin (filling in those wrinkles and sagging skin).
- Improve your muscle tone. (You need this water if you are lifting weights).

How Much Water Should You Drink?

Check with your personal physician first, as this is in no way medical advice. The average person should drink 8 eight-ounce glasses of water a day. And, for every 25 pounds you are overweight, an additional 8 ounces.

Most of my clients carry a water bottle around with them to remind themselves to drink the water. (I know one guy who just fills up a one-gallon container and sips from it throughout the day.)

Oh … coffee is not water. Tea is not water. Juice is not water. Soda … get it? *Water.* Add a slice of lemon, if you want some flavor.

And, one more thing: Stop drinking about three hours before bedtime.

A Review

Step One—Eat to get thin. You need to eat.

Step Two—Get a "B." You only need to succeed at this 85 percent of the time to win!

Step Three—Enjoy it 100 percent! When it begins to become "mindless eating" and you're not enjoying it to the maximum, you are done. Stop.

Step Four—Know when to stop eating. Eat like a small child or a naturally thin person.

Step Five—Exercise Consistently. Aim for *six* days a week.

Step Six—Water, water, water. Drink your water, people!

This is so simple. You can do it!

"This is finally something that worked. I've lost twenty pounds and I'm keeping them off. This also keeps you positive in your life in general and focused at keeping the weight off. If you follow the system, it will work."

—— Brendan Duffy

"I no longer feel out of control with food. I now exercise daily and make better food choices.

"I lost thirty-two pounds and over ten inches from my waist."

—— Jean Griffea

PART 3

Reprogramming Your Life

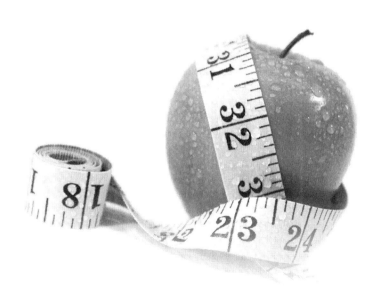

Why You Do What You Do

Did you know there are only two reasons why you do what you do? You can actually sum up almost all of your decisions by these two things.

Pain And Pleasure

The fact is that you only act because of two things:

- Moving towards pleasure.
- Moving away from pain.

That's it. Period. *You desire to seek pleasure or avoid pain.*

You chose to lose weight to avoid pain. Most people who want to lose weight don't really do it to fit into better clothes. Usually it's the pain, both physical and emotional, associated with excess weight that drives one to lose it.

There are some of you who may want to lose weight because you want to look better or feel better, but it's probably (and I am generalizing, of course) the fact that the *pain* of being overweight is causing you to want to move toward the pleasure of becoming thinner. (It's a thin line, really.)

A Sharp Stick

Imagine there's a sharp stick in your back and someone's poking you with it. What will you do? Yes, you'll move away from it.

Poke—move—poke—move.

You're motivated to get thin and you're succeeding.

Poke—move—poke—move.

Getting Thinner... But, You've Plateaued! Why Is That?
Think about it. You've lost twenty or thirty pounds. The pain is less. The stick is dull, like a finger poking you in the back.

Poke—tolerate it—poke—tolerate it.

Now, you're not moving. So, what will you need to do? Yes, *sharpen the stick.*

How do you do this? Increase the pain or pleasure. This is where you will need to create a new reason why you want to lose weight. (Just having the reason of "because I want to" isn't enough.)

Write down *why* you want to lose weight. You're thinner now, so *why* is it even more important to get to your goal?

After successfully losing some weight, do you want to just "tolerate" being twenty or thirty or more pounds overweight? Or, do you want to break through and lose that last amount?

Sharpen the stick. Set down on paper *why* you must do this.

Note: If you skip this part, the potential of backsliding and regressing is possible. Sharpen the stick now!

Last On The List

Let me try to read your mind. (This isn't easy, because you're reading this book and I typed this a while ago. But, assume that I can.) Ready?

You are a caring person who takes care of the world and puts everyone else first. And, for the most part, you are the last on the list.

Did I get it? Now, this isn't so for everyone reading this book—I'm not the Amazing Kreskin, you know. But, for almost 90 percent of my readers, this is a true statement. You put everyone else first and you last.

Believe it or not, this has a name for it: the *Messiah-Martyr Syndrome.*

Savior To Your World

The Messiah-Martyr Syndrome affects many people who are overweight. If you are in a "caretaker" career (nursing, teaching, social worker, physician, etc.) or situation (taking care of elderly parents, children who need assistance, etc.) you may be hostage to the Messiah-Martyr Syndrome.

Even salespeople and entrepreneurs are subject to the Messiah-Martyr Syndrome because they take care of their business or clients first.

So, what is it? The Messiah-Martyr Syndrome is, like I said above, where you put everyone else first and you last.

You take care of the kids, make sure they get dressed, eat,

and get to school. Then the spouse is attended to for a bit. Did you eat breakfast? Probably not because you were too busy running around doing stuff for everyone else!

Then, you get to work and put out fires all day, doing everything for your boss or your business or your clients. You drive someone to the airport or do a "favor" for them. If (and I mean *if*) you eat lunch, you're eating it on the run or at your desk and still working between bites.

You get home and you still have laundry to do, need to pay the bills, drive the kids to their activities, make dinner…

And, by the time you get to what you need to do—you're too pooped to do it.

Exercise? Forget it. I'm too tired now. But, tomorrow—yes, tomorrow I will do better.

Then, you go to bed and repeat it all again.

The funny thing is that everyone else gets *their* needs met. The kids get driven to every sporting event, movie, etc. Your friend gets picked up at the airport. Your boss gets his laundry or coffee. But, what about *your* needs?

You haven't eaten, except for one or two meals. You didn't "have the time" to exercise because that time was sacrificed (messiah) to your list of people's needs and wants.

Put Yourself First

When you travel on an airplane and the flight attendant explains the procedure where if the plane loses pressure and the oxygen masks come down and you have small children seated next to you, whose mask are you instructed to put on first?

No, not the child's—*yours!* Because if you pass out, you both will be gone. You need to put yourself first in this situation.

The same thing applies in life. Imagine for a moment that you've been abducted by friendly aliens from another planet. (Just go with me on this for a bit, okay?) You're on the mother ship looking down at your life. No one knows where you are for days or weeks.

Grieving process aside, *life will go on.* Your kids will get dressed, eat, and get to school. Your spouse will get the laundry done and drive the kids to their activities. Your work will get done by somebody else.

The point is that without you, everything still gets done. But, right now—in your mind—you are the savior to your world (messiah) and you've sacrificed yourself (martyr) to the situation.

What if you put yourself first? Do you know what will happen? Well, here's your epiphany moment:

The actual truth is that even after you've put yourself first, everything on your list of other people's needs will get accomplished!

Yes, it's true. You can take care of yourself first and still do all the things for those people, too. (I'm not asking you to not help them at all; I am just saying you need to put yourself first. That's all.)

This idea is really from an economic rule called *Pay Yourself First.* Briefly, no matter how much money you make, if you "pay yourself first" (sock away thirty dollars each week, for instance), the money will never be missed and your needs will still be met. And, at the end of the year, you'll have a nice savings.

The same thing applies with your life. Replace *Pay Yourself First* with *Put Yourself First*. This will be easy for some and difficult for others.

It's About Time

For some, it's a matter of time management. You will need to set an "appointment" with yourself to eat and exercise and even rest. (Author's Note: If I don't exercise in the morning—first thing—it won't get done. I, personally, need to exercise before I begin my day and I "set an appointment" with myself to do this.)

Others have a bigger situation. You may be a single parent with several kids and two jobs. And, you're taking care of an elderly parent who is living in your house. You begin to *just think* about putting yourself first and you are wracked with guilt.

"But, they need me!" you exclaim. "I *must* do these things for them."

I do totally understand how life can overwhelm someone to the point where you are almost paralyzed. However, the truth is that if you stay fat, overweight, or obese, get sick (diabetes, heart disease, stroke, etc.), or blow out your knees or back … then, *who will be there to take care of those on your list?*

You'll be out of the picture and useful to no one. (Pain. Sharp stick!)

So, somehow, figure out how you can put yourself first. Perhaps, you start small. Train yourself to eat breakfast. Then lunch (sitting and eating, not working and eating).

Then, create an exercise time, before your day begins, and do it consistently—Step Five!

Soon, you'll be in better shape, happier, healthier, and able to help out. Nice, right?

Changing Your State

I know, the title sounds like I suggest that you move out of town to another part of the country to lose weight. (That's not a real practical or workable idea anyway.)

So, what do I mean by "change your state"?

One of the main reasons why people eat comfort foods is to feel better about themselves. It makes you feel better at the time. Food is like a drug. It changes how you feel—just like a drug does. In hypnotism, we call this "changing your state."

Now, you can change your state a number of different ways.

You can:

- Take a powerful narcotic.
- Read a good book.
- Watch a funny movie.
- Eat an apple pie with vanilla bean ice cream!

Of course, that last one is no good because you'll just kick yourself for doing it, rationalize that the weight-loss method you're using isn't working and, well, "…what the heck? Since I blew that diet I might as well eat more! *Right*?"

But, what if you can change your state without using food or drugs? What if you can change how you feel about yourself at the time with … *hypnosis*?

Yes, hypnosis. As a professional certified clinical hypnotist, I've helped thousands of clients improve their lives. And you can, too!

Special Bonus:

As a special bonus for buying this book,
you have the wonderful opportunity to download a
hypnosis program; this is the same hypnosis program
I sell on Amazon.com for thirty-seven dollars!

And it's yours for free.

Go now to this web site:

www.GetThinBeHappy.com/bonuses-book

and follow the easy instructions to download
your FREE hypnosis program!

About Hypnosis

What Is Hypnosis?

Hypnosis refers to the natural state of mind—and of deep, physical relaxation—in which a person becomes highly responsive to suggestions. Hypnosis is not in any way harmful or dangerous. *Every day each and every one of us enters into a hypnotic state quite naturally.*

Am I Aware Of What's Going On Around Me While I'm Hypnotized?

Absolutely! You are quite consciously aware of everything happening around you, just as you would any other time.

Is Hypnosis Dangerous?

This is a question that always comes up. The answer is *no*. Why? Because hypnosis is a totally natural state of mind. You experience it every day when you daydream, remember past events, and even while driving!

No one can ever get "stuck" in a trance; it's 100 percent impossible. (For instance, if the hypnotist were to leave the room, one of two things would happen: [1] Either the person would wake up because they'd realize no one is talking to them; or [2] they would drift into a nice, relaxing sleep and wake up when rested.) If there was an emergency (like a fire, for example), the person would realize what is happening and come out of the trance *instantly.*

What Does It Feel Like To Be Hypnotized?

The answer I get most often is, "I was so relaxed. Now I feel so refreshed." *You know that feeling you get right before you fall asleep at night? That's what it's like.* When you are brought out of hypnosis, you feel refreshed and revitalized like you just had a good night's sleep.

Who Can Be Hypnotized?

Anyone can be hypnotized except someone who is heavily intoxicated, of low intelligence, or unwilling to cooperate. Otherwise, *anyone who wishes to participate can be hypnotized!*

How Can Hypnosis Help Me?

If you wish, hypnosis will help you quit smoking, lose weight, reduce stress, relax for sleeping, improve your golf or tennis game … almost anything you'd like to improve in your life, hypnosis can help improve it.

How Fast Does It Work?

Pretty much … as fast as you'd like. Most persons quit smoking, for example, in one session. However, they must be committed to quitting, not just believing it's a "good idea." Then, one should have some follow-up sessions to reinforce the changes that took place. All you need is a high motivation to change, and the hypnosis can do its work!

More Facts

- Hypnosis heightens your senses; it doesn't "weaken your will."
- The American Medical Association recognized hypnosis as a science in 1958.
- You cannot be made to do anything against your will while hypnotized.
- The more intelligent a person is, the more likely a candidate they make as a hypnosis subject.

- One hour of hypnosis is equal to approximately four hours of sleep.
- The Vatican approved hypnosis to ease pain during childbirth.
- Many athletes use hypnosis to heighten and increase their performance.

Note: The above information represents Bryan Toder and Wizard Marketing Corporation's beliefs based on his experience and professional training and certification. Bryan Toder and Wizard Marketing Corporation assume no liability for any activity entered into as a result of reading this information.

Emotional Eating

Many people say to me that they eat because they are bored, tired, or nervous. They eat to change how they feel. Again, they eat to *change their state*.

Use the free hypnosis program (above) to do this.

And …

I have another way for you to feel better. It's called changing your physiology.

Physiology?

The way you stand, sit, breathe, walk, talk, etc., all contribute to how you feel at any given time. In the hypnosis field of Neuro-Linguistic Programming (NLP) it is called *physiology*.

How To Feel Bad

Want to feel bad? Well, no one does, but try this experiment: Stand up. Look down. Breathe in a shallow way. Slump your shoulders. Move slowly. How do you feel? Kinda blah?

How To Feel Better

Now, try this: stand up tall. Look up. Breathe deeply. Hold your shoulders back. Move about quickly. Feel better? Usually you will.

Changing one's physiology is one of the quickest ways to change your state. If you get some bad news, for instance, your breathing may slow down, you may look down, and move and talk slower than you usually do. The bad news triggers you to change your state and you feel worse than before you heard the news.

So, instead of doing what you've done in the past (which is finding some tasty food to pick up your spirits or drinking a cold beer to feel better), this time change your physiology. It works and it doesn't contain any calories!

Goals And How To Meet Them

Be Careful How You Say It!

Realize that *how* you express what you want will affect the actions you take. Your level of belief is determined by your words—even those you express to yourself in your mind.

Be Targeted

Your goals should be specific. How will you know you've gotten there unless you know what you want in the first place? The way to get on target is to ask yourself the right questions.

Write down your questions and answer them in a confident voice.

Some Sample Questions:

- How will I look when I am thinner?
- Why am I really doing this?
- What *specific* actions do I need to do daily to become thinner?
- What will other people say when I am thinner?

Come up with some other sample questions on your own. Review your answers whenever you need to remind yourself of your commitment to being thin.

Special Bonus Section

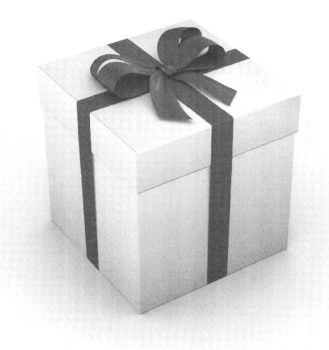

In this Special Bonus Section, I am placing many of the same hypnosis and NLP (Neuro-Linguistic Programming) techniques and exercises that I teach my clients. These exercises and techniques are GOLD. Please value them.

Linking Pleasure To Exercise

"I hate to exercise!"

"It's too hard to do!"

"I don't have enough time!"

"I don't like going to a gym!"

"I'm just not motivated to exercise!"

Face it; you're going to need to exercise. To lose fat and keep it off, exercise is essential. There's no way around it.

So, let's make it fun to do. One of the best ways to do this is an NLP exercise to create a *link* between exercise and pleasure.

NLP, by the way, is the best way to effect change in people within *minutes*. (Seriously, minutes.) The first NLP technique we'll do is:

Creating The Motivation To Exercise

1. Determine where you are now, on a scale of one to ten, where ten is the highest feeling, how motivated you are to exercise. Let's say, for this example, it's a three.

2. Think of a time in your life when you were highly motivated to do something. Perhaps it was going on a trip, meeting someone new, buying a car … whatever. But, be sure to find a time in your life when you were *truly* motivated to do something. This is important.

3. *Visualize* what that time was like. What did you see? Who was there? What colors do you remember?

4. What *sounds* did you hear at the time you were motivated? Perhaps you said things in your head or to yourself to motivate you. What were they? What did other people say to you, or did you overhear someone say something about you?

5. What did it *feel* like to be that motivated? Where in your body did you feel this? In your head? Your chest? Your torso or legs? Was it a cool or warm feeling? Was it steady or did it move around your body?

6. Now, take what you *saw*, *heard*, and *felt* and make them more intense. Make the pictures brighter, bigger, and closer. Make the sounds louder and sharper. Make the feelings stronger.

7. Create a scene or a movie with what you see, hear, and feel. Run the movie forwards and…

8. When the feeling of being motivated is high (a nine or ten), make a tight fist with your left hand and say, "*Yes!*"

9. *Break your state* by looking about, standing up, and sitting down. Just do something to get you momentarily distracted.

10. Next, run the movie again and repeat steps eight and nine. Then, do this one more time.

11. *Testing*: After breaking your state again (just move around or think of the third letter of your middle name), make that tight fist with your left hand and say, "Yes!"

By doing that, you should feel motivated. Do this every time you want to be motivated to exercise; make that tight fist with your left hand and say, "Yes!"

Your Compelling Future

The Dickens Pattern is an NLP technique popularized by Anthony Robbins in his *Unleash the Power Within Seminar*. Tony is an amazing teacher of NLP, and he uses this technique to facilitate quick changes in people and create a compelling future for them!

This pattern is based upon the Charles Dickens' character Scrooge when he meets the Ghost of Christmas Future and is shown the future of what his life will be like if he continues his current behavior and life choices. The pain this causes for Scrooge allows him to make better choices that change his life, and the lives of others, forever.

Remember, we do things because of pain or pleasure. Not exercising enough means there is not enough pain to do it. You won't drink enough water because not enough pleasure is associated to it.

But, let's stay with pain because it's *such* a great motivator! The Dickens Pattern will help you associate pain with *not* doing something, associating consequences with the lack of taking action.

The Dickens Pattern—*What Are the Consequences of Staying the Way You Are Now?* Let's travel forward in time fifteen years.

1. Stand up now in the present. First, it's not as comfortable as sitting and you are changing your physiology.

2. Visualize what your life is like right now. How is your health? Are you fat and overweight? No energy to do

anything? Not motivated?

3. Now, imagine what it would be like to be five years older. And, you haven't done anything to change. But, you *have* changed! Now, you're fifteen pounds heavier. You're fatter and maybe your knees are shot. *What would this cost you in all areas of your life?*

4. Now, you're another five years older, ten since we started, and you're in a wheelchair or walker. You're sick and your back is weak. Walking is almost impossible for you. *What would this cost you in all areas of your life?*

5. Lastly, you are another five years older, fifteen since we started, and you are fatter, sicker, and older. *What would this cost you in all areas of your life?* What a horrible, awful life.

6. Is this what you want? Feel what that would feel like. Imagine what you'd look like in the mirror. What would other people be saying about you? Painful, isn't it? Really associate with those feelings! (The more you feel these feeling and the worse you feel doing this, the better this will work!)

7. Now, imagine it was all a bad dream. Come back to the present. (Better?) *What did not taking action cost you in the future that you imagined?* Your health? Your family? Needless pain and suffering?

8. *Imagine changing the way you do things now.* Make the time to exercise and do it. Eat better. Drink your water. Put yourself first.

9. Associate with the massive pleasure you now have after changing your behavior.

10. Change your physiology: Jump up and down or shake

your body around.

11. Repeat this anytime you get complacent.

That was rough, wasn't it? But, it's one if the best ways to facilitate change in your life!

Trouble Visualizing?

Some people say that they can't visualize pictures in their mind very well. If that's you, can you picture your child's face? Your front door? What color is your car? What does your pet look like and what color is it?

Get the picture? You can visualize.

Controlling Cravings

I love this technique and my clients learn it, use it, and are truly amazed that it works.

Creating A Resource State And Anchoring It

A resource state is simply a state of mind that is useful in a certain situation. Although fear can be useful if you're running from a lion, it's far from useful if you're planning on changing your life.

Accessing a Resource State

Remember when you first fell in love or the last time you felt happy and you'll find that your mood changes. Your mind will begin to duplicate the thought patterns of the positive memory. We want to use this fact to access useful thinking about food and activity.

Remember how a smell can remind you of your mom's kitchen or an aftershave can remind you of your father or anyone from your past? Those memories can come flooding in based on the simplest trigger (or anchor) from our senses.

You can use memory to access positive and secure feelings about anything; however we'll be primarily concerned with feeling full and satisfied with less food.

Creating the Anchor

Step 1: Remember a time after a meal when you were full and satisfied, but not "stuffed." How did you feel? What did you see or hear at the time that you felt full? When did you know that you were full and satisfied?

When the memory is the most clear and as you get a handle on it, you are going to form a physical "anchor" to recall that memory at will. When the memory is in your mind and you have reproduced the feeling of being full, *then touch the back of your ear for about five seconds.*

It is extremely important that you get that "full" feeling. If you don't, you will end up anchoring the feeling of nothing to your ear.

Now, think about anything else; this clears your mind. Repeat Step 1 two more times.

Check to make sure that you feel full when you touch your ear. Congratulations; you have created an anchor.

Step 2: At any time you need to feel full and satisfied, go through the motions of recalling that memory by touching the back of your ear. You will find that you duplicate the impressions in your mind that cause your body to feel more full and satisfied.

Note: Don't confuse the simplicity of this technique for its effectiveness. This is very advanced hypnosis (NLP). Also, *this will not work if you are "famished,"* but you should never get that way.

Here's How To Use The Anchor

Use this anytime you feel a craving for food. For instance, it's late at night and the kitchen is closed. You're watching television and you want something to eat. You're not hungry, but it would be nice …

Then you remember the anchor! You touch the back of

your ear—the same way as you did above—and, ah! You get that "full and satisfied" feeling!

This really does work—if you do it.

Fixing Your Self-Image

In his famous book *Psycho-Cybernetics* plastic surgeon Dr. Maxwell Maltz wrote about his patients who, after being in disfiguring accidents, would have their faces brought back to near perfection through surgery.

Most of his clients went away happy, but he was amazed at the reaction of quite a few of his clients. Even after bringing their faces back to "normal," with no scarring or disfigurement, some of his patients—mostly women— would still see themselves as "ugly."

They were "scarred on the inside," and, no matter what they really looked like on the outside, they could only "see" themselves as disfigured. They had a bad self-image.

Do you have a self-image of always being fat? If so, let's change that! You need to "see" yourself as thinner before you really do become thinner!

For this next exercise, you may want to close your eyes. Read the steps a few times first to get an idea of how they flow and try them with your eyes closed.

Bonus Audio Recording

Go to this website and you can just listen to the
steps in the following exercise!

www.GetThinBeHappy.com/bonuses-book

The "Thinner You" Mirror

Imagine that you can see yourself in a mirror. You are at
the weight, shape, and size you want to be.

See it. Close your eyes and really imagine it. See yourself
wearing that smaller dress or suit. What does that really
look like to you?

Hear what people are saying about you. Listen to what
you are saying to yourself as you look at the mirror and
see the new you!

Now, *step into the mirror* and imagine that you are in the
mirror wearing that dress or suit!

Feel what that new dress or suit feels like on your body.
What does it feel like to have a smaller waist, stronger legs
and arms, or better knees and back?

Imagine going through your daily routines with your new
body. What does that feel like? What do you hear? What
can you see?

Hold onto that feeling. This is the you that you will
become and the you that you are now. This is the new,
thinner you!

"I went to my doctor for my yearly physical...
I am a diabetic and have been for
approximately nineteen years.

"She has reduced my diabetes medication on
one of them and completely taken me off of
another. (The one I was taken off of was one of
the most invasive.

"I had been on four different medications when
I started. I am noticing my blood pressure is
down and I am exercising daily."

— P. Wolf, after just six weeks.

Questions and Answers

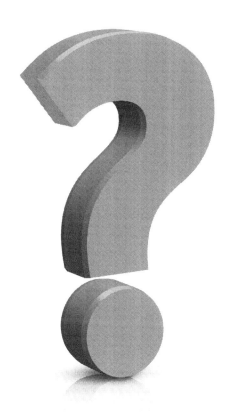

Throughout the years of teaching my clients to lose weight with the techniques in this book and hypnosis, a few questions pop up from time to time.

You haven't told me exactly what to eat! Do you have a diet plan?

No, no, no. Remember, diets do not work. In reality, you already know what to eat. You know not to eat a bucket of fried chicken or burger, fries, and a soda.

Just remember the formula for portions:

A *protein* (poultry, beef, pork, fish) the size of the *palm* of your hand.

A *complex carbohydrate* (brown rice, 100 percent whole wheat bread, potato, etc.) the size of your *fist*.

A *vegetable* a few times a day.

Are all carbs "bad"?

You need carbs in your diet for energy. The mitochondria are the "energy factories" in your cells, and, without getting detailed, you need carbs for energy fuel for the mitochondria.

Remember, too, that you need to eat to maintain your metabolism.

I have heard the terms "simple" and "complex" carbohydrates, but what do they mean?

Imagine you have a large cauldron of water you want to boil over an open fire pit. To boil the water you need fuel. So, you get some logs, some newspaper, and some twigs and light it up. The fire lights and in about fifteen minutes or so, the water is at a nice boiling temperature.

Now, how do you keep it boiling? You simply place some logs (in your case, *complex* carbohydrates) in the fire every so often. If you let the fire go out, you need to start all over again. *However, it only takes a little fuel now and then to keep the water at a boil.*

Imagine that your metabolism is that water and you need to keep it at a boiling point. Do you start skipping meals? No, because the fire will go out and you'll be famished. Your metabolism will remain low, too.

Someone who skips breakfast, has a big lunch, waits until 7:00 PM to eat a huge, clunky dinner and then goes to sleep will just keep getting fat as their metabolism remains at a slow rate.

Skipping meals and then having a bunch of chips or cookies and soda is like tossing a bunch of leaves on the fire; all you'll get is a huge burst of flame that will go out quickly and won't get the water boiling any faster. (This is why when you drink some soda or have some chips you get a tired feeling soon after.)

Eat when you wake up in the morning and eat when you're hungry. *Don't skip meals.* This will keep your metabolism running at a good rate (i.e. keeping the water boiling).

In Step One, I mentioned *complex carbohydrates.* Complex carbohydrates take a long time for the body to burn, like a log on a fire. One hundred percent whole wheat bread (and whole wheat bread, unless it says "100 percent Whole Wheat" isn't whole wheat), brown rice, a potato, etc. are complex carbohydrates. Chips, white bread or rice, pretzels, soda, and the like are simple carbohydrates.

For the most part, avoid eating refined sugar, white flour, and salt. Eat fresh foods, meat, fish, poultry, vegetables, and fresh fruit. Stay away from processed food as these contain more fat, sugar, and salt than most products.

By the way, if you cut out those three sodas a day, you will save about $2,000 a year. Nice!

An Important Note About Fat

Fats are essential in the diet, especially for proper hormonal balance. Dietary fat is also necessary for the absorption of nutrients from fruits and vegetables. It keeps your skin soft and is a great source of energizing fuel.

Reduce excessive fats and eat essential fats.

Eating will not necessarily make you fat. Eating more calories—from fats, carbohydrates, protein, and alcohol—than you burn off leads to weight gain.

At nine calories per gram, fat is calorie-dense. Carbs and protein have only four calories per gram and alcohol has seven calories per gram. (See the next section for more on alcohol.) Since fats are in so many of those tasty foods we love (such as processed foods, fries, chocolate, pastries, ice cream, steak, cheese, etc.), it's easy to overeat fats.

Avocados and olives are not considered veggies, but they are essential fats. Fats from plant sources such as nuts, seeds, and avocados are healthy fats. Flaxseed oil and olive oil are great fats and are wonderful for burning body fat. Omega-3 fatty acids are great too and are found in fatty fish, such as salmon, catfish, mackerel, and trout.

You can get these in capsule form for daily use, but getting them from food is better.

People avoiding fats altogether are generally going to eat carbs that turn to body fat instead. Healthy fats are a critical part of a healthy diet, and avoiding fats actually causes chronic disease.

A good, healthy meal contains approximately 48 percent carbohydrates, 45 percent protein and about 7 percent fats. As you can see, fats are in our diet because they are necessary.

Note: Be careful with cheap salad dressing too, usually found in fast-food chains and restaurants, which may contain soybean oil (a cheap substitute for a better oil) and partially hydrogenated oils which, of course, should be avoided at all costs.

What about alcohol and beer?

Many people think alcohol is sugar; it is not, and it's broken down differently. Since alcohol isn't a carbohydrate, it doesn't offer any energy to the body so it goes directly to the liver, leaving fatty deposits.

Interestingly, women have a different enzyme in the stomach than men, which does not allow them to break down alcohol as quickly or as easily. Additionally, alcohol has a lot of unnecessary calories: seven calories per gram. This isn't an excuse for the men to drink more or women to drink less; it is to inform you that what we consume is broken down and used in the body as fuel.

Food is energy—it has a purpose for more than pleasure. If possible, you should reduce, limit, or avoid alcohol in general *because the calories consumed are providing no nutritional value to the body.*

Is it okay to eat before I go to bed?
It's best to eat no sooner than three hours before you go to sleep.

What happens when you eat late at night before you go to sleep is that you don't get the restorative sleep you need. Instead, *your body is spending it's time and energy digesting the food!*

Your body needs sleep to dream, repair itself, and rest, among other things. If your body is digesting food all night, it can't do that. This leads to sickness, disease, premature aging, and more.

Have you ever eaten a very large meal at night? When you woke up in the morning, chances are you were tired, even after a long night's sleep. The reason is, again, your body spent most of the night digesting food and you, probably, only received a few hours of sleep.

I'm glad I can eat when I'm hungry, but I still feel guilty. Is that okay?
No. Please follow the plan and eat when you're hungry. Stop feeling guilty and make sure you enjoy the food 100 percent. Then *stop* when you are full.

If I fall asleep while listening to the hypnosis program, will it still work?
Yes, everything is heard by your subconscious mind. However, for optimum performance, it's best to listen to the program when you're not so tired (like you are at bedtime, for instance). Listen to the program during some other time of the day.

Can I still lose weight without exercising?

Well, yes, but very little and not for long. As I wrote above, you'll need to exercise consistently to lose fat and to keep it off. *Be sure to check with your personal physician before beginning any weight-loss program.*

I had a great week and then—I blew it! Now what?

Great! You've recognized what you've done. Now, put it behind you and keep going. Do all *six* steps of the *Get Thin—Be Happy!* Program and you'll succeed!

Realize that this is a lifestyle change and things take time. Relax and enjoy the ride.

It's been ten days and I haven't lost any weight!

Hmmm. Weighing yourself, are you? Follow the program and do not weigh yourself.

True story: A client entered my office for her appointment and she was livid. She had just come from her doctor who had weighed her and she was furious. After just five weeks, she'd only lost three pounds.

I just smiled and told her to measure herself when she got home.

The next week, she entered my office waving a small paper and smiling ear to ear. She'd lost inches all over.

Remember: Muscle weighs more than fat. This is a *fat-loss* program and not just weight loss. The weight will come off, but just give this program—and yourself—a chance! You are not in a race. *You are losing the fat slowly, remember?*

Oh, no! I've plateaued! This always happens!

First, you can't say it *always* happens because you've never done this way of losing fat before.

Second, are you really following the program and doing all *six* steps? Are you cheating?

If not, begin to eat more slowly and concentrate on *Step Four: Know When to Stop Eating.* You should break through your plateau!

Note: As most people do, doctors will use the scale to determine if you've plateaued. Remember, since muscle weighs more than fat and you will be gaining muscle as well as losing fat, you may not lose more weight, however, you will lose fat and even a size or two!

I'm going to a wedding and dinner isn't until late. I don't want to spoil my dinner and …

Let me stop you here. Spoil your dinner. Like most families, when we went to an event, my mother would always say, "Don't eat a big lunch! We're going to have a nice dinner and you don't want to spoil it!"

We couldn't snack or anything. Of course, when we arrived we were starving! Apparently, so was everyone else because the poor wait staff was always attacked by the crowds of hungry guests hovering around the kitchen doors.

The food was always greasy and cheesy hors d'oeuvres. By the time we sat down to eat, no one was that hungry, but we still ate.

So, here's what you *should* do: Eat something before you go. Have a small sandwich. When you arrive, forget the hors d'oeuvres and have some fruit. When you eat your meal, follow the Steps!

Then, while everyone is bloated and holding their stomachs, you'll be out dancing!

Final Thoughts

You can do the *Get Thin—Be Happy!* Program easily. You really can. But, you must start.

Some people buy a book like this, read it, and tell themselves that they will "get to it" someday. Of course, that day never arrives.

Now's your chance to change your life! Start the program. Schedule your time. Put yourself first. Eat when you're hungry. Begin to exercise.

You Can Succeed, But It's Up To You

Only you can do this for you. If you need help, however, I am only a click away. Our Web site, www.GetThinBeHappy.com, is packed with tons of helpful videos, audios, and e-books—many of them are free!

As a special bonus, you will have the opportunity to join the *Get Thin—Be Happy!* Community where you can visit online with other program participants on our forum and participate in our TeleSeminars. We usually charge seventeen dollars a month for this, but you'll get this for just one dollar (one dollar!) when you visit our Web site.

ADDITIONAL RESOURCES

We have created some additional resources for your ongoing weight loss success!

Introducing—

The Get Thin—Be Happy! Hypnosis USB Drive

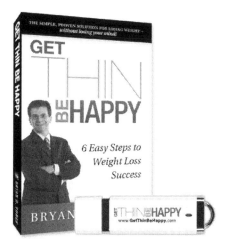

Hypnotist Bryan Toder has created for you several amazing hypnosis programs to help you continue your weight loss success!

To see the benefits of the *Get Thin—Be Happy!* Hypnosis USB Drive, just go here:

www.GetThinBeHappy.com

Life-Changing Skills

As a part of Bryan's hypnosis practice, he has created some amazing audio programs for his clients.

For readers of *Get Thin—Be Happy!* he has made these available to you!

If you've tried to stop snoring before and failed, you can...

...with SnoreBuster:

"Stop Snoring Once-And-For-All With This New Hypnosis CD Program That Will Eliminate Your Sleepless Nights—Almost Immediately!"

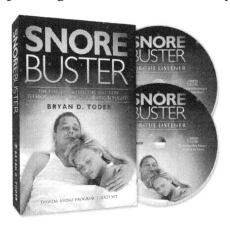

www.BryanToderStore.com

The No Fear Zone Series

Many times, fear causes limited beliefs in people that cause them to become paralyzed in their daily life. Hypnotist Bryan Toder as created a series of audio programs to help you with these fears.

Fearless Speaking—

"Discover The Way to Become A Fearless Speaker That Always Gets The Job, Impresses the Boss And Enjoys The Big Raises & Promotions!"

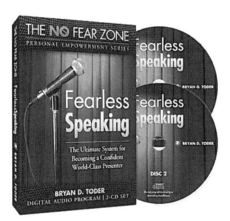

www.BryanToderStore.com

Coming Soon TheNoFearZone.com will include topics such as:

- **Fear of Driving/Driving Over Bridges or Through Tunnels**

- Fear of Bugs/Dogs/Snakes

- **Social Anxiety & Scrutiny**

- Thunderstorms & Loud Noises

- **Fear of Success/Fear of Failure**

- Fear of Flying/Leaving Home/Terrorism

- **Fear of Dentists/Doctors/Needles**

- Fear of Closed Places & Elevators

- **Fear of Woman & Rejection**

… and more!

Just go to TheNoFearZone.com or BryanToderStore.com and see what's new!

New!

Imagine if you had the ability to THINK just like the most successful people in history.

You can. Starting Now!

At last! A fresh approach for taking total control of your financial destiny...

In this 3-volume audio program, Certified Hypnotist Bryan D. Toder you will teach you the **13 Steps Toward Riches**, as popularized by Napoleon Hill in his classic book *Think and Grow Rich*. Best of all, you will discover how to easily apply each of the steps to your everyday life—*Right Now*!

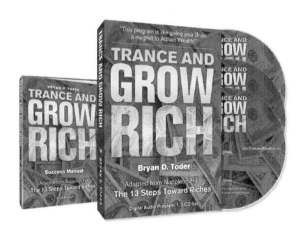

www.BryanToderStore.com

Stop Trying to Play Golf The Hard Way…

"At Last! You Can Lower Your Golf Score And Play Better Golf Than You Ever Have Before—Without A Lot Of Time!"

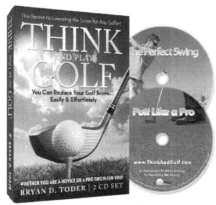

I finally discovered a HIGHLY-EFFECTIVE way to improve my clients' golf game—in just a few days— easily and effortlessly!

It was nothing short of amazing! Of course, it didn't take long before my clients found out about this ground-breaking new secret and asked for my help with their golf game, too.

And the results were astounding! This newly released work called *Think and Golf* is the quickest and easiest way to lower your score. Inside this amazing work you'll get all of the tools you need to mentally master your game. Absolutely everything any golfer would need.

www.BryanToderStore.com

Additional Programs Coming Soon:

- **Quit Smoking**
- Sleep (Get a Great Night's Sleep!)
- **Stress Release & Stress Management**
- Confidence Creator
- **Anger Management**
- Get Organized

...and more!

Just check into www.BryanToderStore.com and see what's new!

Made in the USA
Charleston, SC
16 October 2012